Getting Pregnant

The Essential Guide

How to Conquer Fertility Setbacks and Finally
Have Your Baby

Crystal Sage

ISBN-10: 1514360217
ISBN-13: 978-1514360217

DEDICATION

For those in search of different things they can do to
increase their chances of conceiving and becoming
parents.

CONTENTS

INTRODUCTION

It's a question that's been asked a million times..."why can't I get pregnant?" After spending our youth avoiding this situation it's amazing to see the sheer number of women who are struggling with this problem. Never in our wildest dreams did we stop to consider that one day we would wonder why we cannot get pregnant.

Every day healthy women have difficulty becoming pregnant and find themselves calling fertility clinics or just giving up their dreams of ever becoming parents. Little do they know that there are many different things they can do to increase their chances of conceiving. Once they learn how to increase chances of getting pregnant, they soon find they're on the way to becoming parents and holding their own little bundle of joy. This book is intended to help you get one step closer to that goal.

CHAPTER 1 - FERTILITY: A BETTER UNDERSTANDING

Webster defines fertility as a couple's natural ability to produce offspring. Every human being has the natural ability to reproduce (which is part of our body's reproductive system). Do not confuse fertility with fecundity. Fecundity is all about the actual ability of an individual to reproduce. Someone who lacks fertility is infertile; someone who lacks fecundity is sterile.

The most important thing that anyone who wishes to get pregnant should know is fertility. Women become fertile in the early 20s while men become fertile at the onset of puberty. Men produce a little over 500,000 sperm cells a day while women produce a little over 300,000 egg cells in a lifetime. Men ejaculates more or less 300 million sperm cells during sex, while egg cells mature at an average of one every cycle. Understanding fertility can truly help any couple score their dream of having a baby.

Understanding Men and Fertility

As they say, it takes two to tango. So does getting pregnant. There is no such thing as Immaculate Conception (scientifically speaking that is); therefore, in order to get pregnant, one should understand both male and female fertility. Let us start with male fertility.

Consider the facts mentioned above. On average, a male individual produces 500,000 sperm cells a day. It takes 300,000 million to ejaculate completely, and only a handful (at most 100) of them will successfully travel into the fallopian tube. Out of the 100, it only takes one to make a girl pregnant.

Unfortunately, not everyone is lucky to have strong sperm cells that can survive the travel to the fallopian tube. Some men have difficulty impregnating their spouses because of several factors. According to the World Health Organization (WHO), approximately 10 to 20 percent of all men around the world experience low sperm count. This is mostly caused by the male body's reaction to certain chemicals, exposure to radiation as well as heavy metals (not the music genre) or use of drugs, cigarettes and alcohol.

Pollution is also a factor in low sperm motility. So is heat. Studies show that spending too much time in hot baths, sitting for a long period or wearing tight fitting undergarments elevates the temperature of the testes (where the sperm cells are produced).

Improving sperm count is not as hard as it seems. Sometimes, all it takes is proper diet and exercise. Focus on eating fresh fruits and plenty of greens, coupled with grains, legumes and the likes to help boost fertility.

Maintaining ideal weight is also necessary. One must not be too thin so as to decrease sex drive nor to fat which causes higher body temperatures brought about by excessive fat near your sperm holder (aka testes).

Sperm cell anatomy

Perhaps it is also important for us to understand the anatomy of the little guy behind the pregnancy dream, the sperm. From the Greek word sperma, which means "seed", the sperm is the male reproductive cell. It consists of a head, the mid piece and a tail. The nucleus of the sperm cell is in the head and is the part of the sperm cell that penetrates the female egg.

The middle part contains mitochondria, which produces ATP (short for adenosine triphosphate) that serves as the sperm's energy source as it travels to the woman's womb. Of course, there is the tail, which serves as the propeller guiding the sperm cell in its quest to fertilize the egg. A healthy sperm cell should contain all three parts in order to be a potential fertilizer. Lacking in one of the three can cause a failed pregnancy attempt.

Fertility and Women

Familiar with the saying "your biological clock is ticking"? We often hear this when women reach a certain age still childless. It is a fact that age affects fertility. Scientifically speaking, a woman may have produced egg cells since conception, but only 400 of these will reach maturity. Once all 400 have been used, women will reach a certain period called menopause, which is loosely defined as the cessation or end of her menstrual period.

Female fertility peaks at around early 20s and starts to decline by late 20s with a more significant drop at around age 35. Menopausal stage usually starts around mid-40s and 50s wherein pregnancy might be difficult, if not impossible, to happen.

Egg cell anatomy

Compared to the sperm cell that contains three parts, the egg cell is a cell on its own. It is in fact considered one of the largest cells in the body. It is large enough to be seen by the naked eye. The human egg cell (or ovum) measures around 0.12 millimeters in diameter.

The next chapter focuses on the menstrual cycle. One should remember this very important cycle if pregnancy is the end goal.

CHAPTER 2 - THE MENSTRUAL CYCLE

The menstrual cycle is a cycle of changes that occur naturally in the uterus and ovary. This cycle is an essential part of sexual reproduction, and it is the woman's biological clock, or internal cycle, that guides it. The menstrual cycle times the path of the egg cell as well as the preparation of the uterus for a potential pregnancy. This cycle occurs on a monthly basis until a female reaches menopausal stage – a stage where there is a cessation of menstrual period.

The usual length of the menstrual cycle varies from one woman to another. The shortest cycle lasts for 21 days while the longest is at 35 days. On an average, the usual length of the menstrual cycle is 28 days.

The menstrual cycle particularly the ovarian cycle is divided into three phases. Each phase signifies a path in the life of an egg cell. The first phase is the follicular phase, followed by ovulation and lastly the luteal phase. Let us go through the phases one by one

Follicular phase

At this stage, the ovarian follicles that contain the egg cell mature. Such maturation signifies the readiness of the ovary to release an egg cell. Remember that the body releases only one egg cell per cycle (roughly an egg cell per month). This is when the body initially prepares itself for menstruation. Having sex during this time may not result to a pregnancy since the egg cell has yet to mature (see chapter 3: Timing and Sex).

Ovulation

The second phase of the ovarian cycle happens when the mature egg, which was being prepped earlier, is released from the follicles to the oviduct. Once released from the ovary, the egg travels through the fallopian tube to wait for a sperm cell to fertilize it.

Luteal phase

The third phase of the ovarian cycle is called the luteal phase. At this phase, progesterone and estrogen are released in the body. This means that the egg was not fertilized and thus falls as part of the woman's menstruation. It usually takes 14 days from the time of the ovulation for the body to produce progesterone and estrogen.

Knowing your Cycle

In preparation for pregnancy, a woman should be able to identify her cycle to determine her fertile days. The most common way to do so is to track your first day of menstrual cycle until the first day of your next menstrual period. For example, your first day is March 24 and your next period started April 30. That is equivalent to 35 days, which means you have a 35-day cycle. Some women's cycle vary on a monthly basis (sometimes called as an irregular period).

In this case, one can take the average of at least 3 cycles to determine a regular cycle. For example, month one is 25 days, month 2 is 28 days while month 3 is 21 days. On average, that will be equal to a 25-day cycle.

Regulating Menstrual cycle

Exercise plays an important role in regulating your menstrual cycle. Too much exercise can hinder your cycle. Excessive fat can also do the same. Maintain a healthy weight by proper diet and exercise.

Stress is yet another cause of irregular period. Meditate, relax, or do yoga if possible.

Now that you have identified your cycle, the next step to getting pregnant is having sex, and timing it is very critical if you want to conceive. The next chapter discusses this important step in conquering the pregnancy goal.

Crystal Sage

CHAPTER 3 - TIMING AND SEX

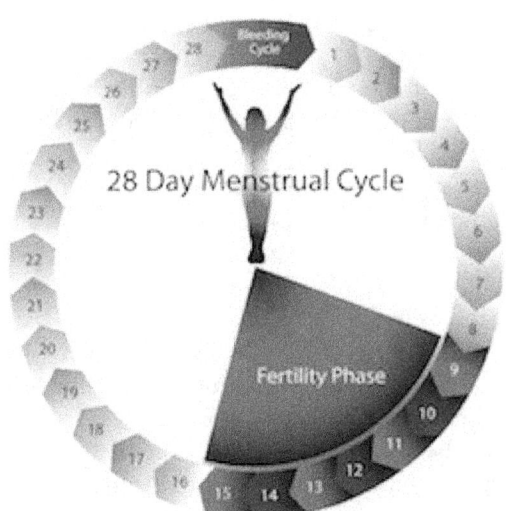

28 Day Menstrual Cycle

Refer to the menstrual cycle above. Credits to www.mayoclinic.org.

One method to determine the perfect time to have sex to increase chances of conception (or avoid pregnancy) is to use the calendar method. In this method, the most fertile period is identified as five days before the ovulation and one to two days after ovulation. On an average cycle of 28 days, this usually is within the 2nd and 3rd week of the menstrual cycle.

Having sex during your fertile period will give a better chance of conceiving.

When to have sex

As they say, timing is everything. An ill-conceived intercourse will not result to pregnancy. To get pregnant, one should have sex as often as possible. A couple having sex more than once a week (at most two to three times a week) will definitely increase their chance of doing it on the woman's fertile day. Sometimes, frequency is all it takes to hit the jackpot.

If having sex often is not possible (conflict in schedule and the likes), make sure that the days that you do have sex count. Consider plotting sex day on your calendar taking into consideration your (or your partner's) menstrual cycle. Here are some tricks to hit the big "O" (in this case ovulation).

Know your cycle

This requires plotting the menstrual cycle for several months. As mentioned, ovulation normally occurs around the 14th day of the cycle and identifying the pattern in your cycle can help you zero-in on an exact day to have sex.

Check that cervical mucus

One telltale sign that you are near ovulation is a noticeable increase in what appears to be slippery and clear secretions in the vagina. You may have to check on this one personally. A "raw egg white-like" secretion is a sure sign of ovulation. After ovulation, the cervical mucus becomes thicker and somewhat cloudy, making it impossible for the sperm cell to penetrate. There are even instances when the cervical mucus disappears altogether – causing dryness down there.

Hot is the new fertile

It is scientifically proven that a slight increase in the basal body temperature indicates ovulation. The basal body temperature is the temperature of your body when you are fully at rest. This may not be determined through ordinary thermometers. You may have to spend some money in order to buy a basal body thermometer, which serves its purpose well. Take your temperature before getting out of bed in the morning and plot your body heat in a chart. You will be most fertile within two to three days before a spike in the temperature arises. A typical increase of around one degree Fahrenheit (equivalent to 0.5 degree Celsius) is enough to imply ovulation.

Ovulation Kit Anyone?

Of course, the advent of technology paved the way for the invention of the easiest solutions to identify ovulation. There are over-the-counter ovulation kits that one can buy to check the level of hormones in the urine. A spike in the hormonal level means ovulation is fast approaching. Make sure to follow the instructions on the label to get the most accurate result.

Is every day Sex the Key?

Although it may sound as if having sex on a daily basis is the key to conception, it is not. In fact, men with low sperm count are prohibited from having sex on a daily basis. The best frequency would be twice or thrice a week. This gives the body ample time to produce sperm cell to fertilize the egg cell. Determining ovulation is not an exact science and engaging in sex two to three times a week gives you a higher chance of getting pregnant.

CHAPTER 4 - WHAT IS YOUR POSITION?

The golden rule for conception is "the deeper the better". In choosing a sexual position where the intention is to conceive, it is advisable to go for one that allows deeper penetration. On top of that, a sexual position that ensures highest orgasm definitely aids the sperm cells in their travel towards the egg cell. The contraption in the reproductive trap brought about by orgasm ensures a smooth sailing travel towards conception.

Here are some sexual positions that may just do that and more:

The Missionary position

This is the most common sexual position and is in fact the most effective means to conceive. To do this position, the woman just needs to lie on her back while the man is on top, doing most of the sexual work.

Why is this effective?

Because the woman's pelvis is not tilted downwards in this position, it helps ensure that the sperm moves closer to the cervix. A man in this position also has a great leeway to achieve a deeper and better penetration. In addition, some say adding a pillow under the woman's hips will help push the sperm further into the cervix.

The Dog-y Style position

This is one of the most common and most favored sexual positions of men. This is a great position not just because of the thrill, but also because it can help couples who want to have a baby. To do this position the woman lies on all fours while the man penetrates her from behind.

Why is this effective?

Penetration is deeper and better in this position and the cervix seemed to be more open compared to others.

The Glowing Triangle Position

This is a variation of the missionary position. To do this, start with a missionary position: the man on top while the woman lies on her back. The only difference is that the man, who is on top, is on all fours while he extends his legs. The woman's hip is raised by placing a pillow underneath her hips. Her legs are also wrapped around the body of the man.

Why is this effective?

This position increases the depth of the penetration while tilting the pelvis of the woman upwards. What makes this better is that the woman is in control. The man needs not move a bit and the woman can do all the work to reach her orgasm before the man shoots of his sperm cells.

The Rock and Roller position

This is also commonly known as the anvil position. This is another variation of the missionary position. Here, the woman is on her back with her man on top. In this position, the woman's leg is raised above her head giving the man a better chance to penetrate deeper.

Why this is effective?

The anvil position targets the G spot of the woman for that come hell and high water orgasm to ensure a better chance of conception.

The Magic Mountain position

This one is a variation of the doggy style although in this position, the woman is on all fours while the man bends over the woman to a point where her back is touching his chest. The woman is bending from the waist down and she uses a pillow for added stability in her upper body. There should be enough pillows to help the women bend her waist in such a way that the pelvis is tilted more than usual.

Why is this effective?

One, it allows deeper penetration. Two, it hits the G spot in the right places. Three, it can stimulate the clitoris for that orgasm, which is definitely ideal for baby making.

Spooning

Spooning is the next most common position, next to the missionary position. In this position, the man is behind the woman as they both lie down in bed.

Why is this effective?

In this position, the pelvis is tilted in such a way that the most number of sperms reaches the cervix.

Orgasm plays an important role in conceiving and if you are an adventurous couple, you might want to try any of the following positions.

Plough position

This may require a complicated stunt called handstand since the woman is literally standing on her hand with her legs up in the air. The man holds the legs of his partner, as if holding a wheelbarrow, and penetrates her from behind.

Why this is effective?

Aside from the thrill of a new position, this position ensures a deeper penetration since the pelvis is directly facing the man.

The Butterfly position

This position requires the woman to lie with her back on a table, instead of on a bed. The man positions himself between her feet. The man holds the woman's legs to raise her hips for deeper penetration of her vagina.

Why this is effective?

This position offers a better penetration as well as the added excitement of the sexual position. The thrill and excitement can make this position more attracting especially for young couples who are still in the process of "experimenting" for love.

Aside from the sexual positions mentioned above another sex trick one should practice is the post sex activity called cuddling. Cuddling is as simple as hugging each other after having sex. Women feel like men don't do much cuddling as they wanted to and for most men the cuddling part feels awkward and unnecessary. Beginning today, remember that if the intent is to get pregnant, then it is important to learn the art of cuddling after sex.

Why is cuddling important?

Scientifically speaking, women release a hormone called oxytocin that somewhat brings out the feeling of wanting to be cuddled. This hormone makes any woman want to bond with her partner. This bond makes her feel ready to have a child. This oxytocin is responsible for keeping any woman's reproductive cycle on track, giving her that biological urge to care for a baby as well as assist in the birthing and lactation process of any mother to be.

Crystal Sage

CHAPTER 5 – WHAT TO EAT AND NOT TO EAT TO GET PREGNANT

In this chapter we will be discussing what types of food one should eat in order to increase the chance of pregnancy. Again, this is about increasing fertility so do not expect that if you persistently eat all the foods mentioned below, it will surely get you pregnant immediately. You do have to wait and see.

Let us start with what you should include in your diet:

1.   *Beans* –
Beans are usually included in the list of fertility boosting foods. According to research made by the Harvard School of Public Health, infertility is found in 39% of their 19,000 respondents. These respondents are recorded to have the highest intake of animal protein. Those who prefer plant protein such as beans find it less difficult to conceive. If the thought of having garbanzos in your salad does not excite you, then you may also add lentils, nuts, or tofu to the menu.

2. *Ice-cream* –

According to a study made by Nurses' Health, a woman who eats at least a serving or two of whole milk as well as whole milk products (such as ice-cream and the likes) have lesser risk of infertility. In fact, those who prefer skim or low fat milk products are more prone to difficult pregnancy. According to theories, the possible culprit behind this is the removal of fat in skimmed or low fat milk.

Less fat causes an imbalance in sex hormones, which results to a difficulty in ovulation. You do not have to sacrifice your diet however. You can replace a serving of non-fat milk with a serving of full fat milk and compensate the extra calories somewhere else.

3. *Green Leafy vegetables* –

Green leafy vegetables have high-level of foliate, which is a B vitamin variant that shows a considerably possible effect on ovulation. Salads such as those made of romaine lettuce, spinach or sides of broccoli and arugula can also be shared with your man since folate is also seen as an effective solution to producing healthier sperm cells.

4. *Pumpkin Seeds* –

These seeds are high in non-heme iron. This iron is in several vegetables as well as iron-fortified foods. Women taking iron supplements (especially those that contain non-heme iron) experience less difficulty in conceiving compared to those non-iron supplement-taking individuals. If taking on supplements seemed costly, then one can go ahead and toast some pumpkin seeds for a crunchy, healthy and definitely worthy snack.

5. *Whole wheat Bread* –

A high-level of insulin is one of the major causes of a disruption in reproductive hormones. Eating complex carbohydrates such as whole wheat bread can help keep insulin (or blood sugar level) stable. According to a study made by several Dutch scientists, women with high insulin level find it difficult to conceive within the 6-month experimental period they set. You can also choose dark bread over white ones or perhaps whole-wheat pasta instead of white ones. This is definitely baby-making foodies.

6. *Olive oil* –

This oil is a type of monounsaturated fat, which causes an increase in insulin activity in the body and in turn decreases inflammation. It is important to avoid inflammation since it is proven to interfere with conception, ovulation, and perhaps the development of the embryo. You can add olive oil to your green salad, or as a replacement for butter when cooking.

7. *Salmon* –

It has been proven that omega-3 fatty acids help regulate reproductive hormones and ensure continues blood flow to reproductive organs in the body. Amongst those fish containing omega-3 fatty acids, it has been proven that salmon has the lowest level of mercury, something that pregnant women and those trying to conceive should avoid.

It is not just about what you eat that is important. One should also focus on what not to eat to protect and increase fertility.

1. *Trans-fats* –

Baked, processed or fried foods should be avoided when one intends to be pregnant. Trans-fats have a tendency to decrease the insulin controlling ability of the body which in turn causes one to be more prone to irregular or erratic ovulation.

Caffeine – no one is stopping you from consuming a cup of coffee a day. You just have to limit it to that level. More than 200 milligrams of caffeine (equivalent to two cups of coffee) can cause major fertility problems. Plus, it can also cause inability to absorb iron, can cause dehydration and in worse case scenarios cause miscarriages.

CHAPTER 6 – BUSTING PREGNANCY MYTHS

For some reason beyond our simple comprehension, myths regarding fertility and getting pregnant have abounded the world. Some may have somewhat scientific basis, but still they do not give the whole story. Others are just simply weird and baseless claims yet many still believe in the truthfulness of such claim. In this chapter, we aim to debunk some of those myths in order to accept truthful ones that definitely serve its purpose.

Pregnancy myth number 1: Orgasm is needed to get pregnant

We may have already discussed in the previous chapters that orgasm may help aid the sperm in travelling towards the fallopian tube but it is not mandatory in every sexual intercourse. In fact, stressing about that big "O" may actually prevent you from enjoying and as they say you have to enjoy it to make it.

Pregnancy Myth number 2: To spit or to swallow?

Another myth is a claim that swallowing your partner's semen can actually increase your fertility. There is no scientific basis for this claim. While it may be true that semen contains a lot of protein, so far no studies have yet to prove that digesting human protein can increase fertility.

Pregnancy myth number 3: Breastfeeding means birth control

This form of natural family planning method is called Lactation Amenorrhea Method (or simply LAM). This requires exclusive Breastfeeding (no other given to the baby) and the mother has amenorrhea and baby is less than six months old to be considered a contraceptive method. Before breastfeeding becomes an effective birth control method, one should look at three things (and all three things should be present to be counted): total lack of menstrual period since delivery of baby (and by total lack it means not even a speck of blood should be present), the baby is fed by breast milk and breast milk alone and that the baby is less than six months old. Considering all of these factors, there is still a 1.2 percent chance of conception. So think again.

Pregnancy myth number 4: Lift those legs baby

The logic behind this acrobatic feat is that lifting your legs up tilts the pelvis and aids the little soldiers to travel the terrain towards the centre of the jungle. As effective as it may sound lifting your legs for more than a minute can actually cause numbness brought about by blood moving away from the feet. Sperms are wired to go find an egg and come hell and high water they will find the way even without you pushing them further. The man sends out more than a million soldiers every battle and a losing a few good men will not hurt the cause a bit. Conception should be fun and not uncomfortable.

Pregnancy myth number 5: Want to have a baby? Forget about booze

This is one myth that is close to reality, but a glass or two shouldn't give you that guilty feeling. A shot or two is not harmful, but going overboard and binge drinking definitely will. Why? Frequent over drinking can result to irregular menstrual cycle which can often time lead to lower chances of getting pregnant since charting a pattern may prove to be difficult to achieve.

Pregnancy myth number 6: Missionary all the way

This one we already have debunked early on (see chapter 4: Position anyone?). Getting pregnant doesn't mean that you can't experiment anymore. The real goal is to penetrate deeper. As long as there is deep penetration and of course ejaculation then there is no problem. Be creative with your styles since time flies when you are having fun. Just make sure to avoid using the lube since studies show it can kill and weaken your man's little men.

Pregnancy myth number 7: One yam equal two babies

What started as a valid research eventually becomes an urban legend with no scientific basis. It was said that a research was conducted in an African village called Igbo-ora where it was recorded that one of the highest rates of giving birth to twins is present. They studied the culture and they found something in common with the parents of twins in the community. They are all fond of eating yams. This started the study linking yams to fertility. This is still in the process so we still have to wait for Harvard Graduate School students to say Yay or Nay for this claim.

Pregnancy myth number 8: Cough syrup + sex equals baby

This one started way back 80s and for some reason still exists up to now. Perhaps it is guaifenesin that should be blamed for this hype. In 1982, a study conducted show remarkable proof of the fertility boosting power of guaifenesin. It has the ability to thin out the cervical mucus in such a way that it thins out the mucus in the nasal passages. If the cervical mucus is thin, the sperm can travel easily to the egg cell. Although it was proven in 1982 it still leaves a lot of question unanswered. For one, cough syrups are not guaifenesin alone. It also contains antihistamine which may have an ill effect towards fertility. Unless you have cough, stay away from cough syrups.

Pregnancy myth number 9: Being on the pill for too long can delay pregnancy

Pills are created to prevent pregnancy although prolonged use of the pill will not stop you from conceiving altogether. In fact, it can actually aid you in conceiving since taking the pills can help you put your menstrual cycle back on track almost immediately. It is seen that women who started on the pill immediately ovulates within the next couple of weeks- provided there are no other issues involved. Studies show that within a year after stopping using pills 80 percent of women do get pregnant. So do not be afraid of the pill.

Pregnancy myth number 10: Adopt a baby and everything else will follow.

Blame Law of attraction for this one. The notion of adopting a baby to conceive a baby is so far one of the craziest myth so far (next to semen ingestion that is) and has no scientific proof to back it up. It may be a coincidence and let's leave it at that.

Pregnancy myth number 11: Prenatal vitamins = conception

Again let us blame the Law of Attraction for this one. Taking a prenatal pill everyday will not increase your chances of getting pregnant any other day. Once you do get pregnant that is the time you take these vitamins to increase the folic acid in your body and to ensure that your baby's spine is protected and strengthened.

There are a lot of myths out there regarding pregnancy and fertility yet one thing is for sure, you need not stress yourself about it. The true key to having a baby is to enjoy the ride. No worries no hassle no stress.

Crystal Sage

A FINAL WORD

Many couple's goal is to conceive a baby and add a little bundle of joy to their household. Some might find it difficult while others do not. You just have to remember a few things:

1. Have sex regularly – to get the highest possible chances of hitting ovulation. Do not overdo it. Twice or thrice a week should do the trick.

2. Avoid stress and strenuous activities – it is all about having fun. The more you worry about something the more it seemed elusive.

3. Be healthy – eat the right kind of food and do a bit of exercise to prepare your body for that day.

4. Know when to seek help- If all else fails perhaps it is time to seek professional help. This does not mean that you are giving up; you are just opening a whole lot of options for you. Do not be ashamed to admit you need help. Do it before it is too late.

Please Leave a Review

Finally, if you enjoyed this book, please take the time to share your thoughts and post a review on Amazon. It'd be greatly appreciated!

That review and feedback will help me improve the content in my books – and make each and every one more relevant and helpful to you.

Thank you again and good luck!

Crystal Sage

www.ingramcontent.com/pod-product-compliance
Lightning Source LLC
Chambersburg PA
CBHW070844290526
45795CB00002B/980